CHAIR YOGA

Improve Your Strength, Flexibility, and Posture
Whilst Creating a Happy State of Mind

OLIVIA BURNS

TABLE OF CONTENTS

INTRODUCTION

Yoga has been practiced for thousands of years by people from all walks of life. Perhaps when you think of yoga, you imagine a mat, some blocks, and people lined up doing the downward dog, and sure enough, that is one way of doing it. However, as with everything, there are plenty of ways to practice an art. Evidently, there is not a "correct" type of yoga. With a little variation, everyone can practice yoga, so long as you find the type that works for you.

Yoga is a practice that began in ancient India. It is a prominent aspect in religions in the Eastern hemisphere, as there is a focus on spirituality and inner life. Yoga is known to be a discipline because it takes a lot of mastering

to clear the mind and feel its benefits. It follows by doing a series of postures in which you focus the mind inside yourself. In

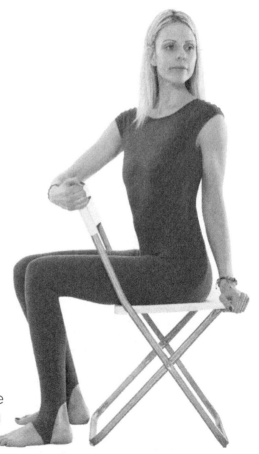

attempts to achieve the postures and clear the mind from external struggles, you will find that you feel much calmer in your day-to-day living. Chair yoga works in the same way. The main difference is that one appeals more to the less mobile. You remain seated in a chair and practice seated postures at the same time as you focus on your breathing and clearing the mind.

Living in an age that is so centered around technology and social media, it's easy to sit down on a couch and not get up for hours. We also live in an age where office jobs are abundant. As easy as it is to sit all day, it is very hard on your body. Because of these factors, many people face issues regarding mobility, energy levels, shortness of breath, a cloudy mind, stress, and more. This means that people of all different ages can benefit from chair yoga! Despite having an evident aid for seniors, there are also clear benefits for kids, teens, and adults who sit on their phones, computers, or other machines all day.

Although cars have been around since the early 20th century, prior to 1945, the idea of everyone owning a single car was foreign (Bronson et al., 2005). This made walking a main mode of transportation to the local spots. Despite it being hard to imagine walking to most places now, it was one of the simple facts of life for most people living before the 20th century. With more people in cars today, especially those who commute far to their jobs (and then proceed to sit at a desk all day), as well as the contributing traffic factor that makes sitting times longer, it can point to the reasons for the decline in the mobility of younger age groups in modern society. Evidently, there are numerous other causes to this decrease in mobility, and the different lifestyles between now and over fifty years ago can be a testament to this.

A study in 2000 was done by The Behaviour Risk Factor Surveillance System (BRFSS) in which a series of questions were asked to two thousand people from all fifty states of the US. To the question, "During the past month, did you participate in any physical activities such as running, calisthenics, golf, gardening, or walking for exercise?" only 26.2% of respondents said, "yes" (Bronson et al., 2005). This number should be much higher, as 30 minutes of exercise should be practiced daily. If you fall into this 26.2%, consider trying chair yoga. Although it's not physically exerting, it will help to get your heart pumping and to stretch out your stiffened muscles.

Whether or not you are a senior citizen, a teen who watches a lot of TV, or an adult who works 9-5 at an office all day, you can benefit from this book! It shouldn't be a negative addition to your life. Rather, chair yoga can bring about positive change to both your physical health and mindset.

It's important to note that everybody is different, and one person's ability is not reflective of everyone's. This book will offer insight, encouragement, and act as a guide into the world of chair yoga. I will touch on the different variations for each pose, which will enable you to pick the posture that challenges you the right way. That being said, this is not an end-all, be-all guide to yoga. You know yourself better than anyone, so take everything at your pace and avoid surpassing your personal limits.

CHAPTER 1
GETTING STARTED WITH CHAIR YOGA

Before heading into the postures, there are a few things you should know beforehand!

WHY CHAIR YOGA?

Chair yoga is much more accommodating to those who struggle with mobility. It doesn't require you to stand up from your chair (unless you are purposefully doing so for a pose). It is a great way to get the body moving even if you have physical issues that can make movement and activity hard.

WHAT YOU WILL NEED

It's all in the name. All you need is (surprise!) a chair. It's really the most convenient form of exercise (or relaxation) because you are able to do it in the comfort of a seat. Ideally, you will need a seat with no arms on it, as there will be some poses that will ask you to stretch your legs to the side or go at the pose from a different side of the chair. Evidently, the type of chair you use is definitely up to you, and if you feel more stable and comfortable with arms at your sides, by all means, go for it!

Other than a chair, it's recommended to be in comfy clothing in order to maximize the movements. Stretchy clothes that are breathable and allow you to move freely are perfect! Another tip is to stay barefoot. This is to maintain a solid grip on the ground in order to avoid slipping on the floor.

GENERAL BENEFITS

There are numerous advantages that come with doing yoga.

- **You can practice chair yoga anywhere.**

As long as there's a chair, there's a way to practice chair yoga! It's as simple as that. If you're stuck in your office working overtime and are just itching to get out of there, take a second for yourself. While staying seated in your chair, you are able to get that break you need without needing to leave the office. The same goes if you're watching a TV show. Even sitting in the passenger's seat of the car, there are postures that you can try out!

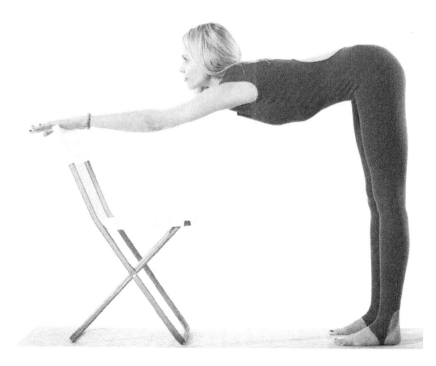

Sitting down doesn't need to mean that you rest. Maximize your sitting time, and use it to your advantage!

· **Get better sleep.**

Because yoga is a meditative practice, it can help to rid the mind of negative or intrusive thoughts that can keep you up late at night. Lying in bed feeling overwhelmed can be very detrimental to your sleep schedule. That's where yoga can come in. Making yoga part of your nightly routine can help to eliminate those stress factors while also bettering your sleep.

Not only mentally can yoga help your sleep schedule, but it is also a physical practice. Because you are using your muscles and moving your body in a way that it doesn't normally, it can make you more tired! One of my favorite feelings is going to bed after a long day of physical exertion, ready for a solid night's rest.

· **Aid and ease stress, anger, sadness, etc.**

Similar to the last one, because yoga can help clear the mind, it can also ease your day's stresses. On average, humans have a maximum of sixty thousand thoughts per day. That is incredibly overwhelming and can cause immense amounts of varying emotion depending on the thought. For that reason, yoga can come in handy. Dedicating a set amount of time to letting go of those worries has been proven to better your mental state. In another study, the International Journal of Yoga wanted to see the importance yoga can have on the mental health of people (Ramanathan et al., 2017). They gave yoga programs to forty elderly inmates, who, twice a week, would get an hour of yoga. The results showed that yoga helped in decreasing significant symptoms of anxiety and depression in adults.

After this study, and much more similar to it, it's now recommended to do yoga of some sort at least twice a week, for a few weeks. If you notice a positive change, keep going, and if you feel it doesn't help you much, perhaps you are looking at the wrong level of yoga.

In the following two chapters, we will look more in-depth at the physical and mental benefits that come with chair yoga.

CHAPTER 2
THE PHYSICAL BENEFITS OF CHAIR YOGA

Despite yoga being a relatively calming practice, it nonetheless is a practice that involves getting the body moving. It isn't the most physically demanding, but it definitely can be tough depending on the posture and your personal mobility abilities. Because it is a physical practice, there are bodily benefits that come along with it! Let's take a look.

BETTERS FLEXIBILITY AND MOBILITY

According to Healthline, "Flexibility is a muscle's ability to lengthen passively, or without engagement" (Walters, 2020). This is why it is incredibly important to maintain good flexibility throughout your life: it limits the number of tears, aches, and pains that you have throughout your life. The more you get your muscles moving, the less pain you will have in response to certain unnatural movements. Of course, it will take a bit of time to get used to this, but in the long run, you will find the postures to benefit you immensely! If you are a senior or someone who sits at a desk all day, chair yoga is a great starting point to work on flexibility. This is because yoga involves moving the body in ways that are not common in everyday living. Moving in these new ways will strengthen your body, making you more flexible and mobile in general. Even those who are active can also strongly benefit from yoga. With such strain on your muscles through sports or other physical exertions, it's important to allow time for the muscles to rest, recover, and regenerate. Your muscles will be able to heal and grow by exercising them softly after a physically demanding day. So, no matter what walk of life you come from, yoga is a great path to take in order to better your body's flexibility and mobility.

BETTERS POSTURE

Maintaining a good posture throughout your life can reduce neck and back pain as well as boost and regulate your blood flow. With this in mind, yoga is a known skill that betters your posture because there is a focus on keeping your back straight and head up. This is because breathing is a necessary center of focus in yoga, and in order to take a full breath in, you must be able to fill your diaphragm, which is best accomplished through a straight seated (or standing) posture. In chapter 5, we will begin with the beginner postures, and you will be able to see for yourself the importance of a straight back.

Working on maintaining that upright position can help drastically improve your posture, as well as master the art of yoga!

STRENGTHENS YOUR HEART

Yoga is all about relaxing the mind and getting your body moving. A combination of these two things is how this practice is known to strengthen the heart. Although you may not be moving too much, you are still getting your blood pumping through your body, and regularly doing so will improve your overall blood flow! Practicing yoga is also known to lower your blood pressure, glucose, and cholesterol levels (The Yoga-Heart Connection, n.d.)! The combination of steady breathing through postures that get your heart pumping is how you are combating future ailments caused by the heart.

CHAPTER 3

THE MENTAL BENEFITS OF CHAIR YOGA

Have you ever been in a high-pressured situation in which you were told by someone else to "take a deep breath?" This is because "deep, slow breathing is associated with calmer states because it helps activate the parasympathetic nervous system" (Harvard Health, 2021). Those deep breaths can help to re-center the mind and concentrate on the task at hand, which is the main idea of yoga!

Although yoga is a physical practice in which you get your body moving, it is also a highly mental practice as well. It works in a way that your mind is able to achieve a higher state of consciousness. You—the yogi—are able to become fully present. What is this mental practice? Meditation.

MEDITATION

Meditation is a fascinating and delicate art in which you find stillness in yourself. It is a process in which you are able to regain peace and focus in your mind. By achieving this state of relaxation, you are able to calm the mind, re-center your day's focus, facilitate breathing, and much more.

Many of the Eastern religions of the world, including Hinduism, Buddhism, Sikhism, etc., utilize components of meditation into their everyday religiosity. This begins the roots of meditation, which is now a universally practiced phenomenon.

By being able to re-center one's focus, you can achieve a lot more in the day. Perhaps you often feel overwhelmed with your long list of things to do. The day is too short, and you have a year's worth of things to achieve in too little time. When it reaches nightfall, you realize that you weren't able to finish everything, making you feel discouraged and like a failure.

Practicing meditation can help you through these moments of stress and hardships. This is because taking a few minutes out of your day to connect back with yourself can help you a ton. I know, I know, it's hard to give yourself some time that's just for you, but it really has proven to help. According to Healthline, after an 8-week study was executed, it was proven that through daily meditation, stress reactions and conditions like inflammation, IBS, PTSD, anxiety symptoms, etc., were all reduced (Thorpe, 2020). They compared two sets of people: one group was getting a Mindfulness-Based Stress Reduction program, which focuses on mental health, and the other was getting a Health Enhancement Program, which focuses on physical health. The results pointed toward more benefits and stress-reduction to come from the first group receiving MBSR.

In another study, 47 people who were all living with chronic pain underwent an 8-week meditation program. They all experienced the benefits of meditation. Their pain lessened and those battling mental illnesses like depression and anxiety reported that meditation bettered their mental states (Thorpe, 2020).

So, you may be wondering, how does this have to do with yoga? Yoga is a great tool in achieving meditation. Without meditation, yoga may have little effect. By incorporating the physical movements of yoga, your busy mind is able to redirect its thoughts to focus on your breathing. When it comes to yoga, the postures aid in this focus on your breath. While your breathing quickens depending on the pose, focusing the mind on taking deep breaths through the nose and out through the mouth will help achieve this meditative state. This centering of focus is the groundwork for meditation. Once you begin to center the mind, you are beginning to reach a deeper state of consciousness. Ultimately the goal of meditation is to become present with yourself. Because we are constantly thinking about the things we have to get done, anticipating future events, or regretting things that have already been done, it's difficult to truly live in the present moment. In order to clear the mind, we must redirect our concentration to something static, like our breathing.

IMPORTANCE TO OTHER ASPECTS OF LIFE

Not only can meditation help you in mastering yoga, but the art of focused breathing and concentration can help you in many other areas of your life as well! For example, whenever you are undergoing a stressful situation, it's easy for your mind to be taken over by irrational thoughts and lots of stress. In this scenario, it's important to stop and take a second to close your eyes and practice box breathing. It can help your rational mind come back out, helping you through the situation that is making you worried or overwhelmed.

The art of meditation can also improve your sleep. After a long day, when you finally get ready to lie down in bed, you may become struck by thousands of thoughts reminding you of all you have to do. This can become very bothersome and stressful, jeopardizing your sleep.

According to Sleep-Foundation, it is recom-mended that adults should receive an average of 7-9 hours every night; however, it's been noted that about 25.2%

of Americans receive less than seven every night (Suni, 2021). One way to help clear the mind at night and get to that recommended target area of sleep is to practice nighttime yoga.

Making this part of your nightly routine will help ease and refocus the mind, getting you ready for a good night's rest.

GETTING THE MOST OUT OF YOGA

Yoga is all about relaxation, revitalization, and rejuvenation. It is a great way to quiet the busy mind. In doing so, it will make you feel brand new mentally. Since it is both a physical and mental experience, yoga is a great way to get active while also working on shifting the day's stresses away from you in times when they aren't needed to be thought about. It enables you to live in the present and focus your concentration on the five senses.

In order to get the most out of yoga, you have to be really willing to try it. It might be hard at first to take the moves seriously or to take those deep breaths in and exhale so loudly that your breath can be smelt a mile away. It'll feel silly to start out, but once you get started, you will understand the benefits of putting your all into it.

Be bold and be confident with it! The worst that can happen is that the pose doesn't suit you well, and you find an alternative that does work! And then you can be bold, confident, and comfortable!

CHAPTER 4

WARM-UP

Before beginning, it's important to prepare your body and mind in order to maximize your comfort and relaxation throughout the practice!

GETTING YOUR BODY READY

Prior to beginning your chair yoga, it's important to get your body physically ready. This is because yoga challenges the body by making you move in ways that are unnatural and abnormal in relation to your everyday life. The best way to do this is to roll out your wrists and ankles. Twist them in circles, getting any cracks or stiffness out of the way early. You can rotate your arms in circles and move your head from side to side as well. These are all great ways to enable your blood to start flowing through your body without exerting yourself too much before the yoga practice.

GETTING YOUR MIND READY

As I'm sure you can tell, a major part of yoga is the mental side that goes along with it. For that reason, it's important not to just jump straight into it. If you have had a very long and overwhelming day and then you suddenly begin to do yoga, it will be hard for you to ignore the events that are at the forefront of your mind. Warming up the mind is thus very important.

To start, take in a deep breath. Throughout this book, I will encourage you to practice box breathing as we go through the poses. Essentially, you are making a square with your breathing. This requires you to take a deep breath in for four seconds and then hold it for four. Release the air for four seconds, and then again, hold for four more. Repeat this as many times as desired. This is a great breathing technique because it can be a great way to transition your thoughts away from your day's stresses. By counting the seconds to each breath, you are consciously diverting your attention away from your day and devoting yourself to the practice that lay ahead.

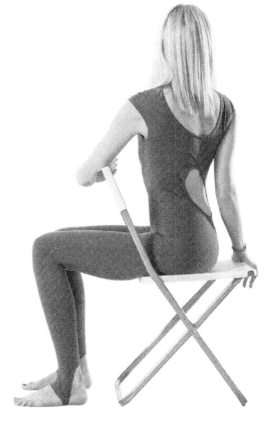

After doing this box breathing for a few minutes, you will find that you are much more relaxed and prepared for chair yoga.

HOW LONG TO HOLD EACH POSE

Since yoga is very breathing-oriented, yogis will hold poses in terms of how many breaths they want to take. On average, it's advised to hold a pose for 3-5 breaths. This can be translated into around 30 seconds to a minute per posture. It's important to work on holding the poses for a period of time because it enables you to focus your attention on breathing and find stillness in yourself. Physically, the best results for stretches come once the muscle has been in a new position for a bit of time because it allows for the muscle to get used to the change. Muscles can get very tight when you don't stretch frequently, so when you do start to, you are actively working on elongating them. The muscle will remain tight until it's been in the position for a while. So, allowing your body time to hold a pose is how to gain the most benefits from yoga.

After you've held the pose for 3-5 breaths, take a moment and come out of your position. Sitting straight up with your eyes closed, take in a deep inhale and let it out. It's recommended to try the posture again once you are ready. You will find that the second time around is much easier. This is because your muscle is now used to being in that position! Over the course of your journey in yoga, you will find that the poses get easier and easier as your muscles become more used to these postures.

READY TO GO

As you go through each posture, remind yourself to focus your attention on your breathing when your mind starts to wander. Ideally, yoga and meditation is a tool to help clear the mind completely; however, we are all human, and that can be incredibly hard to do. When you start to notice your mind wander, bring it back to your breathing and concentrate on your inhalations and exhalations.

As previously noted, yoga is an art that can be practiced by anyone as long as you have the right variations. Each posture or exercise will be explained with two alternative ways to achieve the pose. This is to ensure there is a posture for everyone and that you are able to choose one that works best for you. If you find the posture to be negatively affecting you, or you find you don't feel the stretch, definitely consider the variations. These will include one that lightens the stretch, as well as one that deepens the stretch to accommodate those with different needs. As a starting point, try out the given stretch and see how you feel. Yoga is all about learning about your body and becoming mindful of it, so whatever you need to do in order to achieve that is great!

Remember that it's okay to take breaks! If something is too much for you, try out the variations or take a second to collect yourself and try again. It's important to note that yoga isn't supposed to be painful. Tight muscles can cause discomfort and tension; however, if there's a move that is causing severe pain, definitely stop right away.

CHAPTER 5
BEGINNER'S GUIDE

This chapter will be a great place to start for anyone just beginning chair yoga. This is because the postures won't require much movement around the chair.

This set of postures is ideal for seniors with declining mobility, adults who have major body pains, and those with physical disabilities that limit their ability to get up from the chair. I welcome anyone else to join as well! Remember that there will be variations to each pose in order for you to maximize the stretch.

To get into the posture, we will inhale to prepare our bodies, and then on the exhale, we will come into the full position. Once in the desired pose, hold the posture 3-5 breaths to maximize the benefits to both your mind and body.

As you do each pose, try and keep your eyes closed. This is to allow yourself to concentrate on the movements specifically and limit any visual distractions. A great way to do this is to go through the five senses (with the exception of sight). Take note of what you feel, taste, smell, hear. As you pass through these, you will focus your attention on your surroundings rather than any personal distraction. Focusing on your breath as you do these movements is also an important way to ensure you are getting the most out of yoga.

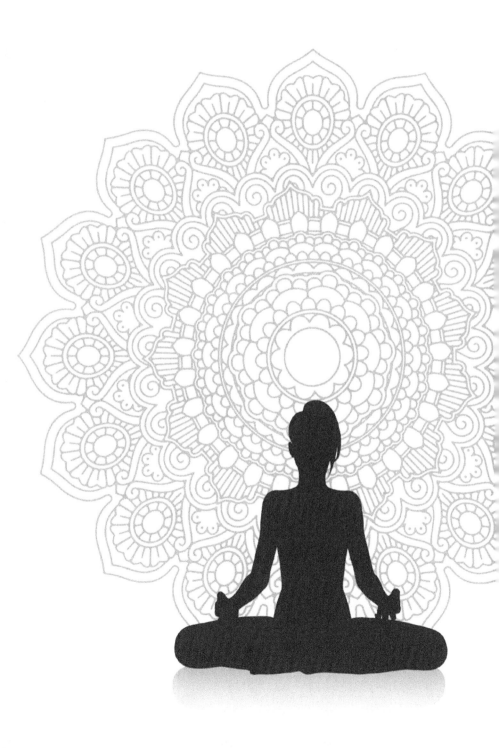

COW AND CAT

This is a classic position in mat yoga and has been made nicely into a pose for the chair!

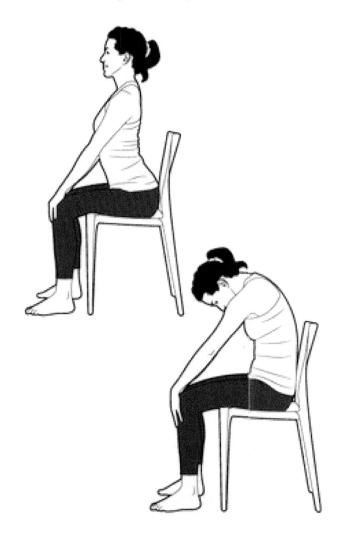

Starting with the cow pose, plant your toes into the ground and feel its energy lift your spine up into a vertical position. Taking a deep breath, arch your back. In a circular movement, bring your shoulders around further behind you. As you exhale, lift your head up, stretching the neck to come into the full pose. Take a few deep breaths here. You should feel this stretch in the shoulders, back, and neck. Make sure to keep your eyes closed in order to maximize the mental meditative state that you are entering.

On your next inhale, round the shoulders back to the front. The back will join your shoulders in rounding the body. Exhaling, lower your gaze to the ground, feeling the stretch in the back of the neck as well as the spine. This is called the cat pose because the rounded back is reminiscent of a cat that's stretching. Hold here for a few breaths.

LIGHTER VARIATION

If the cow and cat posture is too demanding for you at this time, start by just sitting straight up in your chair. Imagine there is a string that's connected at the top of your head, and someone higher than you is pulling on it. Your head will go as high as it can. Really feel this stretch in the back, and let your body become used to the straight-sitting posture.

Focus on your breath and keep your head and help high. After a few breaths, you can try lifting and lowering your head to feel a similar stretch at the base of your neck, like in the cow and cat position.

DEEPER VARIATION

In order to strengthen the cow stretch, try and move your shoulder blades as far back as they'll go. You will feel a stretch of your shoulder blades. If they can't go any further, but you still want to feel a deeper stretch, you can bring your arms out behind you. Taking deep breaths, slowly try to interlock your fingers and forearms, if possible.

For a deeper cat pose, try and round your back as much as possible. You can even lean forward in your chair in order to lengthen the stretch in the lower back.

FORWARD BEND

For this posture, sit only on the front half of the seat. This will provide you with the most mobility and stability throughout the movement.

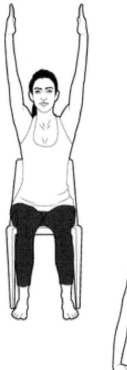

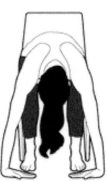

Taking a deep inhale, straighten your back, and bring your hands above your head. You might find that this is challenging to get your arms to reach straight up. This is because we don't tend to lift our arms so high during our day-to-day living. Reach them as far up to the sky as you can and feel it in your upper arms. When you're ready to exhale, bend forward in your chair, coming into your position. Bring your head as far in front of you as you can while keeping your legs in the same position. Allow your arms to hang in front of you, reaching for the ground. Hold this forward bend for 3-5 full breaths. You should feel this pose stretch out your lower back, hips, neck, and shoulders!

Repeat this posture by breathing in and bringing your body back up, reaching your arms to the sky, and then exhaling and releasing your body, folding towards the ground.

LIGHTER VARIATION

If you find this to be so physically demanding that you can't find the relaxation in the pose, you can follow this variation.

Instead of reaching your hands up to the sky, as you take a deep breath in, interlock your fingers and bring your hands to rest on your head. This enables you to feel the same stretch in the same muscle without needing to lift your arms up the whole way. It will still work on separating the shoulder blades and moving them in a way that perhaps isn't done on a regular basis. Make sure to keep your back straight as you inhale.

As you come into the full pose, release your interlocked fingers and move them out in front of you. Here, you can arch the back in order to work on reaching your fingers further from you. This variation will enable you to stretch out your lower back, hips, neck, shoulders, all while not needing to do the complete bend forward.

DEEPER VARIATION

If you didn't quite feel the stretch with the Forward Bend, a way to deepen this stretch is to interlock the fingers and point the palms of both hands toward the sky as you inhale, preparing for the pose. This will rotate your arms, giving you a different type of stretch in the same area near your upper arm. You may also start to feel a stretch in your wrists as you work on keeping your palms to the sky. Make sure you don't lock your elbows as you reach up because this type of hyperextension may cause tissue damage or long-term pain.

On your release, there are two ways you can deepen this forward fold. One allows you to stretch out your legs. Instead of having your legs bent at 90°, stretch them out in front of you. As you bend forward, you will feel a stretch along the back of your leg through the hamstring. Make sure to keep your feet fully planted on the ground. And, similar to the elbows, don't lock your knees for the same reasons. You can also deepen the stretch through the arms. If you can place the palms of your hands on the ground beside you, try bringing them behind you. You can work on keeping your hands flat on the ground or try to reach for the back legs of your chair. This will emphasize the stretch in your shoulder blades, neck, and upper back. Find stillness for a few breaths here.

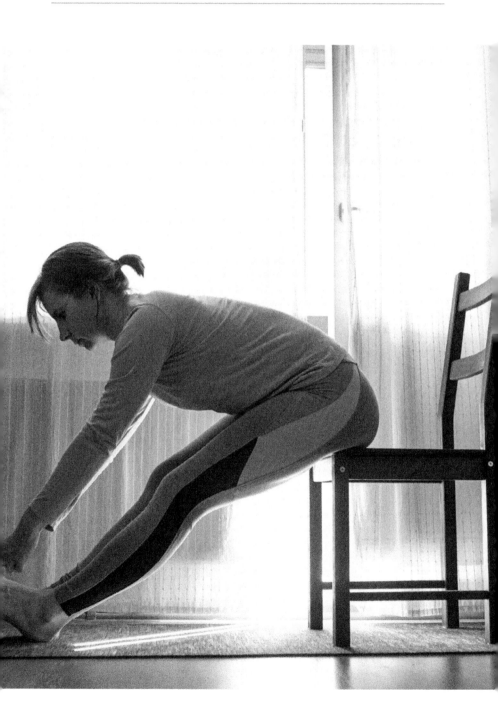

SEATED TWIST

For this pose, rotate your position on the chair so that the back of the chair is at one of your sides. In this explanation, the back will be on your right side.

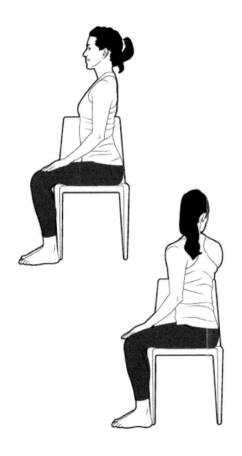

Taking a deep breath in, bring your arms outstretched to your sides and allow them to meet above the head. Keeping the arms straight up, feel the stretch in your upper arms.

As you exhale, turn your body toward the right side. For this, your right arm will bend and rest on the back of the chair, supporting your twist. Let your left arm rest on the outside of your right leg. Being in this twisted position will allow you to feel a deep stretch in your shoulders, as well as every part of your back and hips! Keep your head straight in line with your shoulders as you twist, ensuring that there is no tension there. Remember that this is supposed to be a relaxing pose, so the neck should feel relaxed, too.

Once you've taken the time to find stillness in yourself for 3-5 breaths, remove your right arm from the back of your chair to unravel your twist. Allow yourself a moment of peace by sitting straight up and keeping your head in front of you before trying out the other side.

LIGHTER VARIATION

This pose can be hard to master on your first go, and that's okay! There are plenty of other ways to practice the pose. For a lighter variation, on your inhale, bring your arms up above your head. They can rest on your head if you find that to be more comfortable for you. Hold here and notice the stretch in your upper arms. As you prepare to exhale, release your arms and bring them both to the outside of your right leg. This is instead of reaching your right arm to rest on the back of the chair. Work on getting both the palms of your hands to rest flat around your leg. You should feel the stretch in your lower back and shoulders. You can bring the torso closer to the legs by putting more pressure through your hands to get more out of this variation. Again, ensure that your head is in line with your shoulders and not straining to look somewhere else. Hold this for a few breaths, and then release your arms, bringing them back to rest on the knees of both your legs. Repeat this on the other side!

DEEPER VARIATION

To deepen the seated twist, you can sit on a chair as you normally would. This will help get more out of your twist. As you inhale, if you don't feel the stretch with your arms straight up, try bending them so that the palms of your hands are facing your shoulder blades. This will be felt in your triceps. As you exhale, try and get your arm to rest on the back of the chair as you did when the chair was turned. As you take a couple deep breaths, you should feel your lower and mid-back twist more. If you can, maybe your left arm can grab onto the chair as well and create an even stronger twist. This variation will also open your hips. Keep your head up straight and in line with your shoulders.

Repeat this variation on the other side!

THINGS TO REMEMBER

These poses are perfect for those who are just starting out with chair yoga and have little recent experience with physical activity. In the next chapters, we will look at poses that involve different areas of the body, including the legs, and poses that are slightly harder to achieve. As with these poses, they will have lighter and deeper variations that you can try in order to find the pose that fits you perfectly!

CHAPTER 6
INTERMEDIATE'S GUIDE

For those of us who are more flexible or mobile, you might find that these postures are your perfect fit. These poses will work on all the parts of the body we used in the previous chapter, as well as our legs! Let's look at a few!

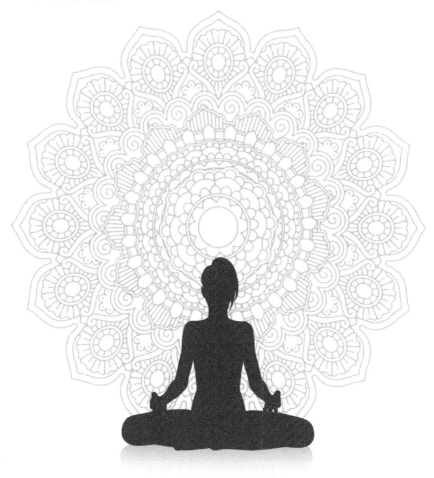

FORWARD FOLD TWIST

This pose involves a mixture of two postures we've already looked at: the Forward Bend and the Seated Twist!

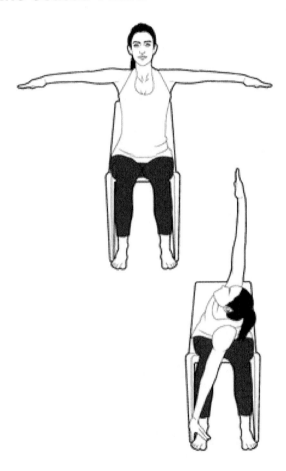

For this one, you will sit near the front of your seat with both your feet planted on the ground. As you inhale, bring your arms out to your sides with your palms perpendicular to the floor. You should feel a stretch in your forearms and inner upper arm as you straighten your arms out. Bring them up over your head, your palms facing the sky.

As you release your breath, twist your body as you bend your upper body forward. The left side of your stomach will meet with your legs, and your left arm will reach for the ground. Keep your right arm pointed at the sky. Your shoulders will open to your right side, making you feel a deep stretch in your arms, hips, back, and shoulders. Take in your deep breaths. Come back to your seated straight posture and repeat this pose on the other side.

LIGHTER VARIATION

To achieve a lighter variation of this Forward Fold Twist, you can sit back further in your chair to get more back support. On your inhale, reach your arms up as high as they go. If you can keep your palms comfortably perpendicular to the ground, try that. If not, place your palms parallel to the ground to get your upper arms stretched out. As you exhale, instead of placing your hands to the ground, try placing your left hand on your right leg and reach your right arm to the sky. Twist your body, bringing your shoulders toward the right side. Your neck and head should follow. Bend your body forward as far as it goes and feel the stretch in your back, hips, and shoulders.

DEEPER VARIATION

If you find that you don't feel the stretch in this pose, you can deepen the move by sitting further back in your chair. This makes your arm stretch farther to reach the floor in front of you, deepening the stretch. As you inhale, you can also reach your lifted arm backward, towards the opposite leg. You will feel a deeper stretch in your bicep and shoulder! As you exhale and come into your forward fold twist, you can achieve a deeper stretch by straightening your legs slightly. While keeping your feet flat on the ground and placing your hand in between your legs, you can feel your hamstrings stretch, achieving a full-body stretch!

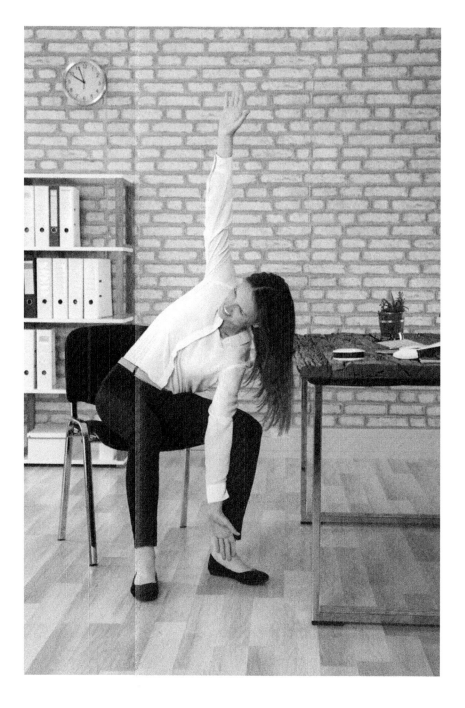

SEATED PIGEON TWIST

For this pose, sit comfortably at the back of your seat.

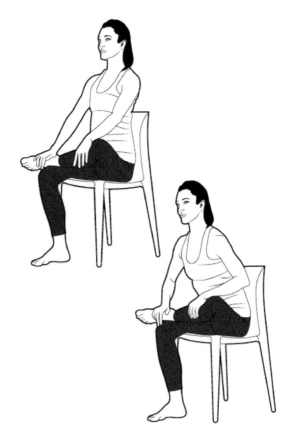

Drawing a deep breath in, grab your left leg up, and have your ankle rest against the thigh of your right leg. You should feel a stretch in your hips as it opens them up. This is a posture in and of itself called pigeon pose, so you can take a few full breaths here before continuing with the rest of the pose.

Next, we are going to go into another twist. Place your left hand on your right thigh and pull against it. Your right arm should reach around toward your lower back on your right side. Your shoulders and spine will naturally turn towards the right side, opening up your chest. Keep your head in line with your shoulders as you exhale steadily. This twist will activate your shoulder and back muscles!

Come back to a straight pigeon pose after you've taken in a few breaths. On your next release, try the twist on your other side, and switch the leg that is folded over to open both sides of the hip!

LIGHTER VARIATION

If this Seated Pigeon Twist is too much all at once, you can try both poses separately. They both will work different muscles in the body, and you will be able to master them separately before trying them together. Another way you can lighten the load of this posture is by crossing your legs as you would if you were sitting at a fancy restaurant. Taking in a deep breath, draw your left leg over your right leg and maintain a strong straight posture. This will still engage the hip, but it won't be as strenuous on the muscle as it would if the ankle were flat on your thigh. On your exhale, you can give the twist an attempt as well. You can make the same variations to your twist by following the Lighter Variations subchapter in the Seated Twist section of the previous chapter.

DEEPER VARIATION

In order to deepen this stretch, try this variation out. On your inhale, keep your torso upright. Instead of having your ankle resting on your opposite leg, try getting your calf to your opposite leg. You can help get this part of the leg to your side by pulling your bent foot toward your torso. You will lengthen the stretch in your hip. Alternatively, you can keep your ankle resting on your opposite thigh, but with one hand, push your bent knee towards the ground. This will also help to lengthen the stretch in the hip.

As you exhale into your twist, you can try reaching your arm further behind you. If you can, reach for the opposite side of the chair and twist your body further by putting pressure on that arm. Keep your head up and avoid craning your neck.

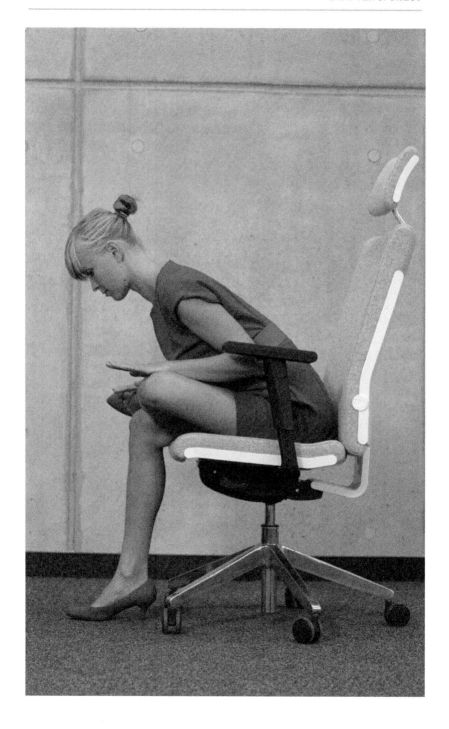

DOWNWARD DOG

Downward dog is a famous yoga pose that I'm sure everyone knows about. It essentially mimics how a dog looks while stretching.

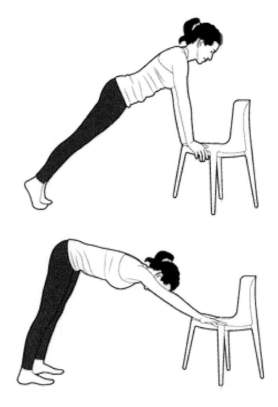

For this pose, you're going to start by standing up and facing your chair straight on. Take a deep breath in through the nose to stand up straight. Find your balance in your stance and hold your peace for a moment.

When you're prepared to exhale, bend your body forward to reach for the base of the chair. Slowly walk your feet away from you until the desired stretch has been achieved. In mat yoga, your hands would be touching the ground, but this is a more accessible way to achieve the pose. Find balance and stillness in the pose and relax your body for 3-5 breaths. You should feel the stretch in your hamstrings, calves, hips, and shoulders. Drop the neck down to the floor, keeping it relaxed. Try to avoid putting tension or strain on the back by focusing your weight on your feet. For this pose especially, you want to make sure your body weight is in your feet. This is because the chair could slide if you put too much weight in your hands. If you are having trouble with sliding, you can place a heavy book or another object on the seat to keep it from moving.

LIGHTER VARIATION

If this posture is difficult for you, consider this lighter variation. Instead of having the chair facing you, you can flip it backward so that the back of the chair is facing towards you.

As you inhale into the pose, find a moment of calmness as you take in your surroundings through your senses. When you are prepared to exhale, place your hands at the top of the backside of the chair and find your downward dog posture from there. Keeping your hands at a higher level will lighten the bend you feel in your legs and shoulders. For this move, too, be aware of the type of chair you use, as placing your weight on the back of a chair can cause it to tip over, which can lead to injury. Be mindful of how your weight is distributed, and aim to have it in your feet. If it's more comfortable for you, add weight to it, or find a sturdier chair.

DEEPER VARIATION

To deepen this downward dog in your shoulders, you can flip the chair as you would for the lighter variation. As you move into your downward dog position, bring your head as low as it can go. Having your hands start at a higher point can deepen the stretch when you move further down. Keep your neck and head loose and relaxed in order to feel the best coming out of this pose. You will feel a deeper stretch in your shoulders.

If you want to deepen the stretch in the legs, you can try lifting one of your heels off the ground while in the downward dog position. In doing so, it will dig the opposite heel further into the ground, and you will feel a deep stretch in your calf. Remember to keep your weight on your feet to avoid slipping or tipping the chair. Take turns switching sides, or you can pulse and switch each time.

THINGS TO REMEMBER

Although these are considered to be at the intermediate level, everyone has very different strengths from the next person! Although you may be around the same level, for someone else, they might find one pose harder than you did and vice versa. Each pose will take practice to master, but with a little time, you will find that they hurt less, and you have become much more flexible, balanced, and mobile! Once you feel comfortable with these postures and have tried the deeper variations, you can try out some of the advanced postures that are explained in the next chapter.

CHAPTER 7
ADVANCED GUIDE

These postures are great for those who have been doing chair yoga for a while and are trying to get a deep stretch out of it. For example, We will be working on all parts of the body, with a focus on balance. As always, there will be variations to make the posture lighter or deeper that you can follow, depending on your skill and comfort level.

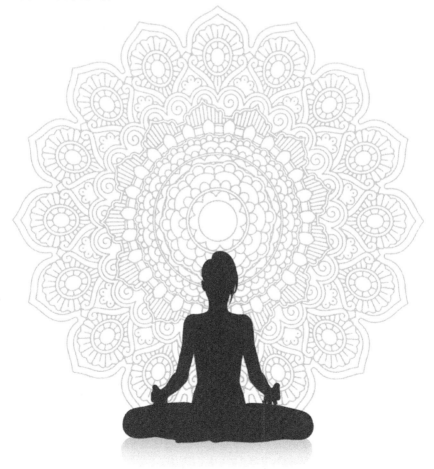

FOOT TO SEAT POSE

For this pose, begin by standing a few feet away from your chair.

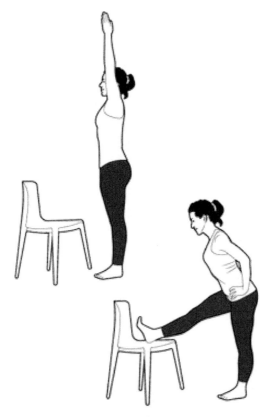

On your inhale, bring your hands up, reaching for the sky. You've mastered this inhale by now, I'm sure. Remember to keep your body straight and your head forward. When you are ready to exhale, bring one of your legs up and rest the heel of your foot on the base of the chair. You will feel a deep stretch in your calf and hamstring. Bring your torso and hands down to rest on your shins or any other part of the leg that feels comfortable. Make sure that as you bend down to meet your leg that you keep your torso straight. Imagine that there is a long piece of wood attached to your back, preventing it from bending. This pose helps to open up the hips in addition to being a stretch for the back of the leg and shoulders. Take in 3-5 deep breaths. When you are ready, return the lifted foot back to the ground and try out the same stretch on the opposite side. Again, make sure that you keep your spine straight when going up and down.

LIGHTER VARIATION

If this posture is too demanding, follow this variation. Inhale normally, reaching your arms up to the sky. As you prepare to come down into position, instead of placing the heel of your foot on the chair, try resting the arch of your foot at the edge of the chair. In order to prevent the chair from sliding, you can rest the chair against a wall or place something heavy on it to keep it in place. By placing the arch of your foot at the edge of the chair instead of the heel on the top, it doesn't flex the foot as much. This creates a lighter sensation at the calf while still enabling the body to feel a stretch in the hips, hamstrings, and shoulders!

DEEPER VARIATION

If you want a deeper stretch with this posture, you can try going on your knees. You can get a soft pillow, blanket, or mat to go under you if it's hard on your knee caps. Starting with your knees on the ground, a few feet in front of your chair, inhale and lift the arms up. As you prepare to exhale, lift one leg up and place your heel on the base of the chair. This deepens the stretch at the back of your leg and also opens your hips more. You can pulse here and try to get your bottom as low to the ground as it can. Don't forget to take in a few deep breaths here!

WARRIOR I

For this pose, we will essentially be making a lunge over the chair.

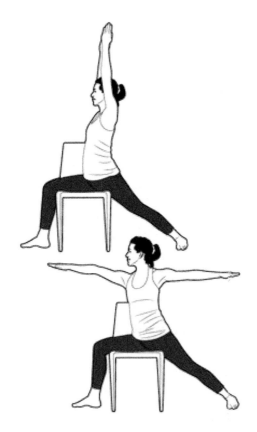

Start by sitting sideways on your seat so that the back of the chair is to one side. For this example, the back of the chair will be on your right side. Instead of having both your feet in front of you, though, place your right foot pointed straight in front of the chair and your left foot behind, getting into that lunge position. Lift your left heel off the ground to keep you the most stable and comfortable. Shift your body so that your right thigh is resting on the base of the seat. Keep your hips pointed straight in front of you, and keep your gaze forward. Depending on the position of your hips, your shoulders will follow, so make sure to keep them squared to help your head stay straight ahead. Bend the torso forward to lengthen the stretch in the hips and shoulders. Point your arms straight in front of you and feel your core tighten. After taking a few breaths, come out of the pose. Take a break and when you are ready, repeat the pose on the opposite side so that your right leg is now extended behind you.

LIGHTER VARIATION

If this pose is too physically demanding, you can lighten the stretch by keeping your back leg bent. This way, more of your weight will be distributed between your legs, rather than having a focus be on the back leg. On your inhale, reach your arms up, tightening your core and keeping your focus forward. As you exhale, instead of leaning forward, you can bring your hands to your heart's center. Do this by putting your palms together and resting them in the middle of your chest. This will work on your balance and core strength.

DEEPER VARIATION

If you are looking to deepen this posture, you can follow the instruction in the inhale as you would for the original pose. As you prepare to exhale, instead of folding forward, tilt your body backward, opening your chest up to the sky. Tilt your gaze upward, following the direction of your hands, and take deep breaths here. You can bring your palms together to try and find balance here. This variation will work on lengthening the stretch in your core, legs, hips, and arms, all while working on your flexibility. If you find you're unsteady, you can bend your back leg to place more of your weight on the chair. If that's too easy, try lifting away from the chair to practice your balance.

BACKWARD BEND

For the final posture, we will try a backward bend.

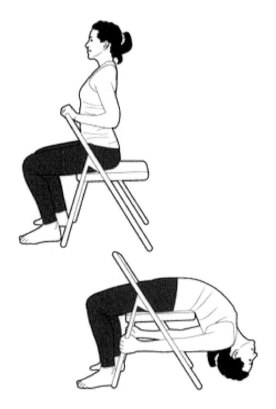

There are many different ways to do this, so feel free to do your own variation to achieve maximum comfort. For today, we will look at three different ways to achieve this posture successfully. For this one, start by having your chair pointed sideways like the Warrior I pose. So, the back of the chair will be to your side. Next, place your upper back on the bottom of the chair so that your stomach is facing the sky. Bend your legs so that the bottoms of your feet are planted to the ground. This is the pose! You should feel the stretch at the backs of your arms and your lower stomach. You can let your head relax over the edge of the chair to disengage the core and neck muscles in order to feel the most relaxed as you take a moment to breathe deeply and meditate.

LIGHTER VARIATION

This pose can be quite overwhelming. If you want to achieve a similar backward bend without needing to place your back to the base of the chair, you can sit on your chair normally. Shift your body so that you are sitting at the edge of the seat. On your inhale, practice the cow posture that we looked at in chapter 5. As you exhale, reach both your arms near the back of the chair. You can grip the chair anywhere your hands reach behind you and arch your back. This will lift the chest out and stretch out your core. Shift your gaze upward and find stillness here.

DEEPER VARIATION

To deepen this posture, try and sit further down on your chair so that your lower back is now being supported by the base of the chair rather than your upper back. This will naturally drop your back closer to the ground. As you exhale, reach your arms straight out in front of you, moving your gaze along with it. Place your weight into the chair as you deepen the stretch in your arms. If you are very flexible, you position yourself into a full backbend, in which the palms of your hands are flat on the floor. Otherwise, adjust your body so that you can comfortably relax in the position while feeling a deep stretch in the back, arms, and neck.

THINGS TO REMEMBER

Although these are considered harder chair yoga positions, like mentioned in the previous chapter, everyone will have their own opinion! Remember to listen to your body—it knows you best!

CHAPTER 8
COOL DOWN

Evidently, there are countless more chair poses that you can work on and master in the realm of yoga, but I outlined a few of the main ones that range from great starting places to the harder ones that take longer to master. Although yoga is not supposed to be too strenuous on the body, it does work to get your heart rate up and blood flowing. For that reason, it's important to give yourself a bit of time to cool down.

SAVASANA

Many yogis will do what's called Corpse pose or the Sanskrit word: Savasana to mark the end of their yoga. This is because it is a very relaxing pose that enables you to focus on meditating. For chair yoga, we will be a corpse that can sit in a chair!

For this pose, take a deep breath in, and let your body straighten itself. Place your palms to your knees, grounding your feet on the floor. With your chin up, draw yourself up as high as you can. Keep your back against the chair to keep your body in line. Find stillness in this pose and focus on your breathing. Work on your box breathing as you come to peace with yourself.

NAMASTE

A common word we say before moving on with our days is Namaste. This is a Sanskrit word that means "I bow to you." It is often used as a greeting; however, in yoga, it ends the practice. We say it to give thanks to ourselves and others for participating. So, before saying Namaste, thank yourself for doing what you did. Thank yourself for being kind to your body. Tell yourself that you are strong, capable, and powerful. You are amazing.

CONCLUSION

You did it! You are on your path to becoming a master chair yogi. How does it feel?

This book has looked at reasons why yoga is important, which includes (and isn't limited to):

· Better Sleep

· Better Posture

· Better Balance/Stability

· Better Flexibility

· Better Mobility

· Stronger/healthier heart

· Fewer aches and pains

· Becoming more present

· Meditation

· Lessening anxiety and depression symptoms

As you can see, yoga is very good for both our mental and physical selves. Whether you are just starting out or have been practicing yoga for a while, there is a posture that you will be able to do. It is very accommodating to all levels and ages, making this art versatile and suitable for everyone.

It's so easy to get caught up with everything happening in the world. We become more stressed, scared, overwhelmed, and sad people by letting our emotions take over. Yoga enables us to take a step and focus on the present moment. Focusing on our breathing and being able to redirect our thoughts away for a certain amount of time is a very useful practice that we can use in our everyday lives. Mastering yoga means mastering meditation, and you don't need to be doing yoga to meditate. When you are about to enter a job interview, a first date, a big exam, etc., take a step back, focus on your breathing and clear your mind. You will become instantly less worried about what the future has to hold, and you will be able to live more presently and peacefully.

Give yourself a pat on the back for giving chair yoga a try! You are actively bettering your body and mind. Good luck on your path to mastering the art of chair yoga.

Namaste.

REFERENCES

Anand, P. (2020, August 14). Chair Yoga for Seniors: 7 Poses To Support Mobility | Snug. Snug Safety. https://www.snugsafe.com/all-posts/chair-yoga-for-seniors

Antanaityte, N. (n.d.). Mind Matters: How To Effortlessly Have More Positive Thoughts | TLEX Institute. TLEX Institute. https://tlexinstitute.com/how-to-effortlessly-have-more-positive-thoughts/#:%7E:text=Tendencies%20of%20the%20mind&text=It%20was%20found%20that%20the,to%2060%2C000%20thoughts%20per%20day

Brownson, R. C., Boehmer, T. K., & Luke, D. A. (2005). DECLINING RATES OF PHYSICAL ACTIVITY IN THE UNITED STATES: What Are the Contributors? Annual Review of Public Health, 26(1), 421–443. https://doi.org/10.1146/annurev.publhealth.26.021304.144437

Chair Seated Twists Yoga | Yoga Sequences, Benefits, Variations, and Sanskrit Pronunciation. (2020, November 4). Tummee.Com. https://www.tummee.com/yoga-poses/chair-seated-twists

Harvard Health. (2019, September 25). The importance of stretching. https://www.health.harvard.edu/staying-healthy/the-importance-of-stretching

Harvard Health. (2021, June 12). Yoga for better mental health. https://www.health.harvard.edu/staying-healthy/yoga-for-better-mental-health

Head Down Chair Yoga (Seated Forward Fold Pose on Chair) | Yoga Sequences, Benefits, Variations, and Sanskrit Pronunciation. (2020, November 3). Tummee.Com. https://www.tummee.com/yoga-poses/head-down-chair

Kovar, E. (2015, June 18). Chair Yoga Poses | 7 Poses for Better Balance. Ace Fitness. https://www.acefitness.org/education-and-resources/lifestyle/blog/5478/chair-yoga-poses-7-poses-for-better-balance/

Link, M. R. S. (2017, August 30). 13 Benefits of Yoga That Are Supported by Science. Healthline. https://www.healthline.com/nutrition/13-benefits-of-yoga#TOC_TITLE_HDR_6

Pitko, C. (2021, May 2). 5 Chair Yoga Poses for All Ages and Practice Levels. DoYou. https://www.doyou.com/5-chair-yoga-poses-for-yogis-of-all-ages-and-practice-levels-57559/

Pizer, A. (n.d.). 10 Yoga Poses You Can Do in a Chair. Verywell Fit. Retrieved August 11, 2021, from https://www.verywellfit.com/chair-yoga-poses-3567189

Ramanathan, M., Bhavanani, A. B., & Trakroo, M. (2017). Effect of a 12-week yoga therapy program on mental health status in elderly women inmates of a hospice. International journal of yoga, 10(1), 24–28. https://doi.org/10.4103/0973-6131.186156

Suni, E. (2021, February 8). Sleep Statistics. Sleep Foundation. https://www.sleepfoundation.org/how-sleep-works/sleep-facts-statistics

The Yoga-Heart Connection. (n.d.). Johns Hopkins Medicine. Retrieved August 11, 2021, from https://www.hopkinsmedicine.org/health/wellness-and-prevention/the-yoga-heart-connection

Thorpe, M., MD PhD. (2020, October 27). 12 Science-Based Benefits of Meditation. Healthline. https://www.healthline.com/nutrition/12-benefits-of-meditation#2.-Controls-anxiety

Walters, M. (2020, July 9). Why You Don't Need to Be Gumby: Mobility vs. Flexibility. Healthline. https://www.healthline.com/health/exercise-fitness/why-you-dont-need-to-be-gumby-mobility-vs-flexibility#Flexibility-vs.-mobility

Warrior Pose I Chair Variation Yoga (Virabhadrasana I Chair Variation) | Yoga Sequences, Benefits, Variations, and Sanskrit Pronunciation. (2020, October 16). Tummee.Com. https://www.tummee.com/yoga-poses/warrior-pose-i-chair-variation

Waterstone on Augusta. (2020, December 23). The Benefits of Chair Yoga. https://www.waterstoneonaugusta.com/the-benefits-of-chair-yoga/

What does namaste mean (2019, January 13). Namaste Meaning. YOGATEKET. Yogateket. https://www.yogateket.com/blog/namaste-meaning-what-you-need-to-know

Williams, S. (2021, March 31). Top 15 Chair Yoga Poses That Anyone Can Practice. YOGA PRACTICE. https://yogapractice.com/yoga/chair-yoga-poses/

Wilson, K. (2015, September 16). How to Avoid Hyperextending Elbows in Yoga Poses. DoYou. https://www.doyou.com/how-to-avoid-hyperextending-elbows-in-yoga-poses-99723/

Printed in Great Britain
by Amazon

46478365R00037